The sir

Cookbook

The essential and tasty Sirtfood Diet recipe book. A quick start guide to cooking on the Sirtfood Diet! Easy and delicious recipes to burn fat and lose weight

By Vilma J. Hernandez

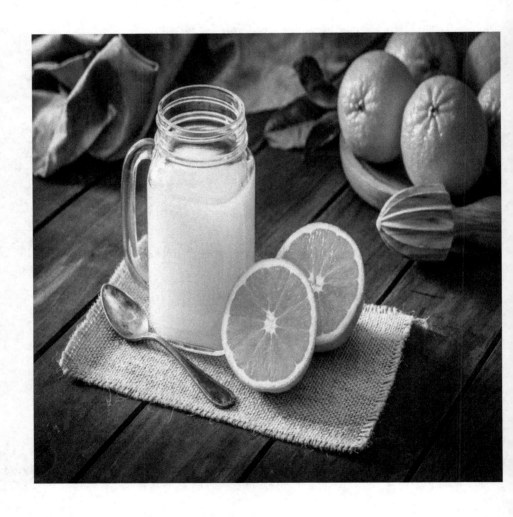

Table of Contents

INTRODUCTION 9

CHAPTER 1. SNACKS 14

1. CELERY AND RAISINS SNACK SALAD 14
2. DILL AND BELL PEPPERS SNACK BOWL 16
3. SPICY PUMPKIN SEEDS BOWL 18
4. APPLE AND PECAN BOWLS 19
5. ZUCCHINI BOWLS 20
6. CHEESY MUSHROOMS 22
7. MOZZARELLA CAULIFLOWER BARS 24
8. CINNAMON APPLE CHIPS 26
9. VEGETABLE AND NUTS BREAD LOAF 27
10. EASY CRACKERS 29
11. ALMOND CRACKERS 31
12. MONKEY TRAIL MIX 33
13. GRANOLA WITH QUINOA 35
14. MED-STYLED OLIVES 37
15. ROASTED CHICKPEAS 39
16. BAKED ROOT VEG CRISPS 41
17. LEMON RICOTTA COOKIES WITH LEMON GLAZE 44
18. PEANUT BUTTER SNACK BALLS 47

19. MASCARPONE CHEESECAKE WITH ALMOND CRUST 48

20. PIZZA KALE CHIPS 51

21. TUSCAN BEAN STEW 53

22. CHOCOLATE NUT TRUFFLES...55

23. CHOCOLATE BALLS..57

24. VANILLA CRÈME BRULE..58

25. HEALTHY COFFEE COOKIES...60

26. STRAWBERRY OATMEAL BARS...63

27. PARSLEY CHEESE BALLS 66

28. BAKED KALE CHIPS 68

CHAPTER 2. SAUCES & DIPS..71

29. SWEET AND SAVORY CHERRY COMPOTE.....................71

30. CILANTRO LIME SAUCE...73

31. GREEK TZATZIKI SAUCE 75

32. GREEN ENCHILADA SAUCE 77

33. JALAPENO PINEAPPLE AIOLI 79

34. AWESOME SAUCE 81

35. VEGAN HOLLANDAISE SAUCE...83

36. VEGAN CHEESE SAUCE 85

37. TERIYAKI SAUCE 87

38. THAI PEANUT SAUCE 89

39. TASTY VEGAN GRAVY 91

CHAPTER 3. JUICES & SMOOTHIES 94

40. KALE KIWI SMOOTHIE 94

41. SALAD SMOOTHIE 96

42. AVOCADO KALE SMOOTHIE 98

43. KALE BANANA APPLE SMOOTHIE 100

44. KALE CUCUMBER APPLE SMOOTHIE 101

45. GRAPEFRUIT KALE SMOOTHIE 103

46. PEAR CILANTRO SMOOTHIE 104

CONCLUSION 105

Introduction

The basis of the sirtuin diet can be explained in simple terms or complex ways. It is essential to understand how and why it works, however, to appreciate the value of what you are doing. It is also necessary to know why these sirtuin rich foods help you maintain fidelity to your diet plan. Otherwise, you may throw something in your meal with less nutrition that would defeat the purpose of planning for one rich in sirtuins. Most importantly, this is not a dietary fad, and as you will see, there is much wisdom in how humans have used natural foods even for medicinal purposes, over thousands of years.

To understand how the Sirtfood diet works and why these particular foods are necessary, we will look at their role in the human body.

Sirtuin activity was first researched in yeast, where a mutation caused an extension in the yeast's lifespan. Sirtuins were also shown to slow aging in laboratory mice, fruit flies, and nematodes. As Sirtuins' research proved to transfer to mammals, they were examined for their use in diet and slowing the aging process. The sirtuins in humans are different in typing, but they essentially work in the same ways and reasons.

There are seven "members" that make up the sirtuin family. It is believed that sirtuins play a significant role in regulating certain functions of cells, including proliferation (reproduction and growth of cells), apoptosis (death of cells). They promote survival and resist stress to increase longevity.

They are also seen to block neurodegeneration (loss of function of the brain's nerve cells). They conduct their housekeeping functions by cleaning out toxic proteins and supporting the brain's ability to change and adapt to different conditions or recuperate (i.e., brain plasticity). As part of this, they also help reduce chronic inflammation and reduce something called oxidative stress. Oxidative stress is when there are too many cell-damaging free radicals circulating in the body, and the body cannot catch up by combating them with anti-oxidants. These factors are related to age-related illness and weight, which again brings us back to how they work.

You will see labels in Sirtuins that start with "SIR," representing "Silence Information Regulator" genes. They do precisely that, silence or regulate, as part of their functions. The seven sirtuins humans work with are SIRT1, SIRT2, SIRT3, SIRT4, SIRT 5, SIRT6, and SIRT7. Each of these types is responsible for different areas of protecting cells. They work by either stimulating or turning on certain gene expressions or reducing and turning off other gene expressions. It essentially means that they can influence genes to do more or less of something, most of which they are already programmed to do.

Through enzyme reactions, each of the SIRT types affects different cells responsible for the metabolic processes that help maintain life. It is also related to what organs and functions they will act.

For example, SIRT6 causes the expression of the genes in humans that affect skeletal muscle, fat tissue, brain, and heart. SIRT 3 would induce an expression of genes that affect the kidneys, liver, brain, and heart.

If we tie these concepts together, you can see that the Sirtuin proteins can change the expression of genes, and in the case of the Sirtfood Diet, we care about how sirtuins can turn off those genes that are responsible for speeding up aging and for weight management.

The other aspect to this conversation of sirtuins is the function and the power of calorie restriction on the human body. Calorie restriction is merely eating fewer calories. It, coupled with exercise and reducing stress, is usually a combination of weight loss. Calorie restriction has also proven across much research in animals and humans to increase one's lifespan.

We can look further at the role of sirtuins with calorie restriction and using the SIRT3 protein, which has a role in metabolism and aging. Amongst all of the effects of the protein on gene expression (such as preventing cells from dying, reducing tumors from growing, etc.), we want to understand the impact of SIRT3 on weight for this book.

As we stated earlier, the SIRT3 has high expression in those metabolically active tissues, and its ability to express itself increases with caloric restriction, fasting, and exercise. On the contrary, it will express itself less when the body has high fat, high-calorie-riddled diet.

The last few highlights of sirtuins are their role in regulating telomeres and reducing inflammation, which also helps prevent disease and aging.

Telomeres are sequences of proteins at the ends of chromosomes. When cells divide, these get shorter. As we age, they get shorter, and other stressors to the body also will contribute to this. Maintaining these longer telomeres is the key to slower aging. Also, proper diet, along with exercise and other variables, can lengthen telomeres. SIRT6 is one of the sirtuins that, if activated, can help with DNA damage, inflammation, and oxidative stress. SIRT1 also helps with inflammatory response cycles that are related to many age-related diseases.

Calories restriction, as we mentioned earlier, can extend life to some degree. Since this and fasting are a stressor, these factors will stimulate the SIRT3 proteins to kick in and protect the body from the stressors and excess free radicals. Again, the telomere length is affected as well.

some people's beliefs, genetics, such as "it is what it is" or "it is my fate because Uncle Joe has something..." through our own lifestyle choices. To what we are exposed to, we can influence action and changes in our genes. It is quite an empowering thought, yet another reason you should be excited to have a science-based diet such as the Sirtfood diet is available to you.

Having laid this all out before you, you should be able to appreciate how and why these miraculous compounds work in your favor to keep you youthful, healthy, and lean To sum up, all of this information also shows that, contrary to. If they are working hard for you, don't you feel that you should do something too? Well, you can, and that is what the rest of this book will do for you by providing all the SIRT-recipes.

Chapter 1. Snacks

1. Celery and Raisins Snack Salad

Preparation time: 15 minutes

Cooking time: 0 minutes

Servings: 4

Ingredients:

- ½ cup raisins
- 4 cups celery, sliced
- ¼ cup parsley, chopped
- ½ cup walnuts, chopped
- Juice of ½ lemon
- 2 tablespoons olive oil
- Salt and black pepper to the taste

Directions:

1. In a salad bowl, mix celery with raisins, walnuts, parsley, lemon juice, oil, and black pepper and toss. Divide into small cups and serve as a snack.

Nutrition:

Calories: 150

Carbs: 30g

Fat: 4g

Protein: 2g

2. Dill and Bell Peppers Snack Bowl

Preparation time: 15 minutes

Cooking time: 0 minutes

Servings: 4

Ingredients:

- 2 tablespoons dill, chopped
- 1 yellow onion, chopped
- 1-pound multi-colored bell peppers, cut into halves, seeded, and cut into thin strips
- 3 tablespoons extra virgin olive oil
- 2 and ½ tablespoons white vinegar
- Black pepper to the taste

Directions:

1. In a salad bowl, mix bell peppers with onion, dill, pepper, oil, vinegar, and toss to coat. Divide into small bowls and serve as a snack.

Nutrition:

Calories: 25

Carbs: 5g

Fat: 0g

Protein: 1g

3. Spicy Pumpkin Seeds Bowl

Preparation time: 5 minutes

Cooking time: 20 minutes

Servings: 6

Ingredients:

- ½ tablespoon chili powder
- ½ teaspoon cayenne pepper
- 2 cups pumpkin seeds
- 2 teaspoons lime juice

Directions:

1. Spread pumpkin seeds on a lined baking sheet, add lime juice, cayenne, chili powder, and toss well. Put it in the oven and roast at 275 degrees F for 20 minutes. Divide into small bowls and serve as a snack.

Nutrition:

Calories: 150

Carbs: 3g

Fat: 13g .Protein: 8g

4. Apple and Pecan Bowls

Preparation time: 15 minutes

Cooking time: 0 minutes

Servings: 4

Ingredients:

- 4 big apples, cored, peeled, and cubed
- 2 teaspoons lemon juice
- ¼ cup pecans, chopped

Directions:

1. Mix apples with lemon juice and pecans in a bowl and toss. Divide into small bowls and serve as a snack.

Nutrition:

Calories: 78

Carbs: 13g

Fat: 2g

Protein: 1g

5. Zucchini Bowls

Preparation time: 15 minutes

Cooking time: 20 minutes

Servings: 12

Ingredients:

- Cooking spray
- ½ cup dill, chopped
- 1 egg
- ½ cup whole wheat flour
- Black pepper to the taste
- 1 yellow onion, chopped
- 2 garlic cloves, minced
- 3 zucchinis, grated

Directions:

1. In a bowl, mix zucchinis with garlic, onion, flour, pepper, egg, and dill and stir well. Shape the mix into 12 portions with small bowls' help and arrange them on a lined baking sheet.

2. Grease them with some cooking spray and bake at 400 degrees F for 20 minutes, flipping them halfway. Serve at room temperature as snacks.

Nutrition:

Calories: 108

Carbs: 15g

Fat: 3g

6. Cheesy Mushrooms

Preparation time: 15 minutes

Cooking time: 20 minutes

Servings: 5

Ingredients:

- 20 white mushroom caps
- 1 garlic clove, minced
- 3 tablespoons parsley, chopped
- 2 yellow onions, chopped
- Black pepper to the taste
- ½ cup low-fat parmesan, grated
- ¼ cup low-fat mozzarella, grated
- A drizzle of olive oil
- 2 tablespoons non-fat yogurt

Directions:

1. Heat-up a pan with some oil over medium heat, add garlic and onion, stir, cook for 10 minutes and transfer to a bowl.

2. Add black pepper, garlic, parsley, mozzarella, parmesan, and yogurt, stir well, stuff the mushroom caps with the mix.

3. Arrange them on a lined baking sheet and bake in the oven at 400 degrees F for 20 minutes. Serve.

Nutrition:

Calories: 181

Carbs: 1g

Fat: 16g

Protein: 9g

7. Mozzarella Cauliflower Bars

Preparation time: 15 minutes

Cooking time: 20 minutes

Servings: 12

Ingredients:

- 1 big cauliflower head, riced
- ½ cup low-fat mozzarella cheese, shredded
- ¼ cup egg whites
- 1 teaspoon Italian seasoning
- Black pepper to the taste

Directions:

1. Spread the riced cauliflower on a lined baking sheet and cook in the oven at 375 degrees F for 20 minutes.

2. Transfer to a bowl, add black pepper, cheese, seasoning, and egg whites, stir, spread into a rectangle pan, and press well on the bottom.

3. Introduce in the oven at 375 degrees F and bake for 20 minutes. Let it cool and slice into 12 bars. Serve at room temperature as a snack.

Nutrition:

Calories: 319

Carbs: 34g

Fat: 17g

Protein: 7g

8. Cinnamon Apple Chips

Preparation time: 15 minutes

Cooking time: 2 hours

Servings: 4

Ingredients:

- Cooking spray

- 2 teaspoons cinnamon powder

- 2 apples, cored and thinly sliced

Directions:

1. Arrange apple slices on a lined baking sheet, spray them with cooking oil, and sprinkle cinnamon on it. Put it in the oven and bake at 300 degrees F for 2 hours. Divide into bowls and serve as a snack.

Nutrition:

Calories: 140

Carbs: 20g

Fat: 7g

Protein: 0g

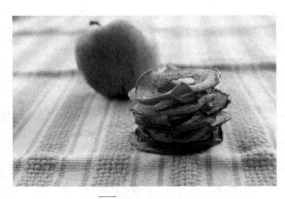

9. Vegetable and Nuts Bread Loaf

Preparation time: 15 minutes

Cooking time: 1 hour & 35 minutes

Servings: 4

Ingredients:

- 6oz mushrooms, finely chopped
- 3½ oz haricot beans
- 3½ oz walnuts, finely chopped
- 3½ oz peanuts, finely chopped
- 1 carrot, finely chopped
- 3 sticks celery, finely chopped
- 1 bird's-eye chili, finely chopped
- 1 red onion, finely chopped
- 1 egg, beaten
- 2 cloves of garlic, chopped
- 2 tablespoons olive oil
- 2 teaspoons turmeric powder
- 2 tablespoons soy sauce
- 4 tablespoons fresh parsley, chopped

- 100mls (3½ Fl oz) water

- 60mls (2fl oz) red wine

Directions:

1. Warm oil in a pan and add the garlic, chili, carrot, celery, onion, mushrooms, and turmeric. Cook for 5 minutes. Place the haricot beans in a bowl and stir in nuts, vegetables, soy sauce, egg, parsley, red wine, and water.

2. Grease and line a large loaf tin with greaseproof paper. Spoon the batter into the loaf tin, cover with foil and bake in the oven at 375F for 60-90 minutes. Let it stand within 10 minutes, then turn onto a serving plate.

Nutrition:

Calories: 83

Carbs: 16g

Fat: 2g

Protein: 2g

10. Easy Crackers

Preparation time: 15 minutes

Cooking time: 60 minutes

Servings: 72 crackers

Ingredients:

- 1 cup boiling water
- 1/3 cup chia seeds
- 1/3 cup sesame seeds
- 1/3 cup pumpkin seeds
- 1/3 cup Flaxseeds
- 1/3 cup sunflower seeds
- 1 tablespoon Psyllium powder
- 1 cup almond flour
- 1 teaspoon salt
- ¼ cup coconut oil, melted

Directions:

1. Preheat your oven to 300 degrees F.

2. Add listed fixing except coconut oil and water to the food processor and pulse until ground. Transfer to a

mixing bowl, then pour melted coconut oil and boiling water, mix.

3. Transfer mix to prepared sheet and spread into a thin layer. Cut dough into crackers and bake for 60 minutes. Cool and serve as needed as a snack.

Nutrition:

Calories: 180

Carbs: 28g

Fat: 5g

Protein: 4g

11. Almond Crackers

Preparation time: 15 minutes

Cooking time: 20 minutes

Servings: 40 crackers

Ingredients:

- 1 cup almond flour
- ¼ teaspoon baking soda
- 1/8 teaspoon black pepper
- 3 tablespoons sesame seeds
- 1 egg, beaten
- Salt and pepper to taste

Directions:

1. Warm your oven to 350 degrees F. Line two baking sheets with parchment paper and keep them on the side.

2. Mix the dry ingredients in a large bowl and add egg, mix well and form a dough. Divide dough into two balls. Roll out the dough between two pieces of parchment paper.

3. Cut into crackers and transfer them to the prepared baking sheet. Bake for 15-20 minutes. Repeat until all the dough has been used up. Leave crackers to cool and serve as needed.

Nutrition:

Calories:

130

Carbs:

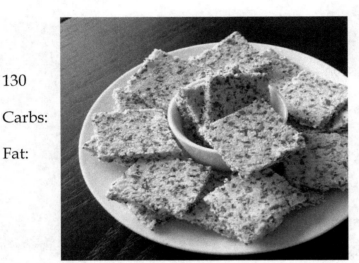

5g

Fat:

11g

Protein: 6g

12. Monkey Trail Mix

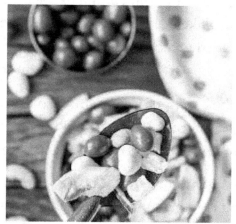

Preparation Time: 1 hour

Cooking Time: 30 minutes.

Servings: 5

Ingredients:

- 1 teaspoon of vanilla extract

- 3 tablespoons of coconut oil

- 1/3 cup of coconut sugar

- 6 oz. of dried banana

- ½ cup of dark chocolate chips

- 1 cup of coconut flakes, unsweetened

- 1 cup of cashews, raw and unsalted

- 2 cups of walnuts, raw and unsalted

Directions:

1. Add the coconut oil, vanilla extract, coconut sugar, coconut flakes, and nuts into a crockpot. Stir to combine, then cook on high for 1 hour. Stir occasionally to make sure the coconut flakes do not burn.

2. Turn the crockpot temperature to low and continue to cook for another 30 minutes. Put the batter out onto parchment paper and allow to dry completely.

3. Allow the mixture to cool before adding the banana and chocolate chips. Store in an airtight container and enjoy when hungry.

4. Use a combination of raw, unsalted nuts to extend the recipe — this can include Brazil nuts or almonds.

Nutrition:

Calories: 151

Fat: 10g

Carbs: 13g

Protein: 4g

13. Granola with Quinoa

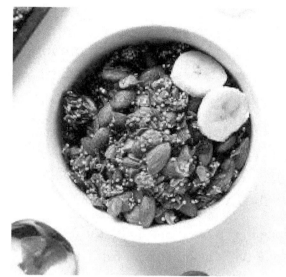

Preparation Time: 30 minutes

Cooking Time: 20 minutes

Servings: 6

- 1 pinch of salt

- ¼ cup of maple syrup

- 3 ½ tablespoons of coconut oil

- 1 tablespoon coconut sugar

- 1 cup of rolled oats

- 2 cups of almonds, raw and unsalted

- ½ cup of quinoa, uncooked

Directions:

1. Warm your oven to 340 F and line a baking tray with parchment paper. In a large mixing bowl, add the salt, sugar, oats, almonds, and quinoa and set aside.

2. In a small saucepan over medium heat, add the maple syrup and coconut oil. Using a whisk, stir until combined, then remove from the heat.

3. Pour the syrup over the mixed nuts and quinoa and give it a thorough stir. Place the mixture onto the baking tray and, using a spatula, spread the ingredients evenly over the dish.

4. Place in the oven and bake for 20 minutes. Remove the tray, give it a shake, and return to the oven to bake for another 10 minutes or until the mixture has turned a golden, brown color. Allow to cool, then serve.

Nutrition:

Calories: 241

Fat: 6g

Carbs: 33g

Protein: 15g

14. Med-Styled Olives

Preparation Time: 10 minutes

Cooking Time: 10 minutes

Servings: 6 servings

Ingredients:

- 1 pinch of salt
- 1 pinch of black pepper
- 1 ½ tablespoon of coriander seeds
- 1 tablespoon of extra-virgin olive oil
- 1 lemon
- 7 oz. of kalamata olives
- 7 oz. of green queen olives

Directions:

1. Crush the coriander seeds using your pestle and mortar and set aside. Using a sharp knife, cut long, thin slices of lemon rind and place them into a bowl with both the green queen and kalamata olives.

2. Squeeze the juice of one lemon over the top of the olives and add the olive oil. Add the salt, pepper, and coriander seeds, then stir and serve.

Nutrition:

Calories: 477

Fat: 9g

Carbs: 60g/Protein: 35g

15. Roasted Chickpeas

Preparation Time: 10 minutes

Cooking Time: 40 minutes

Servings: 6 servings

Ingredients:

- 1 pinch of salt

- 1 pinch of black pepper

- 1 pinch of garlic powder

- 1 teaspoon of dried oregano

- 2 tablespoons of extra-virgin olive oil

- juice of 1 lemon

- 2 teaspoons of red wine vinegar

- 2 15 oz. canned chickpeas

Directions:

1. Warm your oven to 425 F and place a sheet of parchment paper onto a baking tray. Drain and rinse the chickpeas, then pour them onto the baking tray. Spread them evenly.

2. Place them in the oven and roast them for 10 minutes. Remove from the oven, give the plate a firm shake, and then return it to the oven for a further 10 minutes.

3. Remove from the oven and set aside. Add the remaining ingredients into a mixing bowl. Combine well, then add the roasted chickpeas.

4. Using a spatula ensures that the chickpeas are evenly coated. Return the chickpeas into the oven and allow to roast for 10 minutes. Remove them from the oven, allow to cool, then serve.

Nutrition:

Calories: 323

Fat: 15.6g

Carbs: 39.5g

Protein: 10.4g

16. Baked Root Veg Crisps

Preparation Time: 10 minutes

Cooking Time: 30 minutes

Servings: 2

Ingredients:

- 1 pinch of salt

- 1 pinch of black pepper

- 1 pinch of ground cumin

- 1 pinch of dried thyme

- 1 teaspoon of garlic powder

- 2 tablespoons of extra-virgin olive oil

- 1 parsnip, finely sliced

- 1 turnip, finely sliced

- 1 red beet, finely sliced

- 1 golden beet, finely sliced

- Ingredients for the dipping sauce:

- 1 pinch of salt

- 1 pinch of black pepper

- 6 tablespoons of buttermilk

- 1 cup of Greek yogurt

- 1 teaspoon of honey

- 1 teaspoon of lemon zest

- 2 cloves of garlic, minced

- 2 tablespoons of fresh, flat-leaf parsley, minced

Directions:

1. Combine all of the dipping sauce ingredients into a medium mixing bowl, using a whisk to ensure that the sauce is evenly combined. Set aside in the refrigerator for when needed. Preheat your oven to 400 F.

2. In a small mixing bowl, combine the seasoning, herbs, and olive oil. Rinse your root vegetables and dry them off using a kitchen towel.

3. Remove all the root vegetable skins, gently use a mandoline slicer, and slice the vegetables into thin crisps.

4. Brush each side of the crisp with the olive oil and then place onto an oven-proof wire rack. Place the wire rack onto a baking sheet.

5. Bake for 20 minutes or until the vegetables have crisped up. Allow to cool or enjoy them warm with the sauce.

Nutrition:

Calories: 457

Fat: 31g

Carbs: 33g

Protein: 12g

17. Lemon Ricotta Cookies with Lemon Glaze

Preparation Time: 20 minutes

Cooking Time: 15 minutes

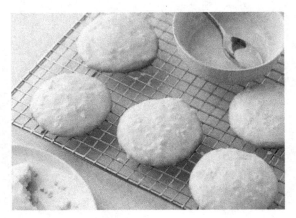

Servings: 44

Ingredients:

- 2 ½ cups all-purpose flour
- 1 tsp baking powder
- 1 tsp salt
- 1 tbsp unsalted butter softened
- 2 cups of sugar
- 2 eggs
- 1 teaspoon (15-ounce) container whole-milk ricotta cheese

- 3 tbsp lemon juice

- zest of one lemon

Glaze:

- 11/2 cups powdered sugar

- 3 tbsp lemon juice

- zest of one lemon

Directions:

1. Warm oven to 375 F. In a medium bowl, combine the flour, baking powder, and salt. Set-aside.

2. From the big bowl, blend the butter and the sugar. With an electric mixer, beat the sugar and butter until light and fluffy, about three minutes. Put the eggs one at a time, beating until incorporated.

3. Insert the ricotta cheese, lemon juice, and lemon zest. Beat to blend. Stir in the dry ingredients — line two baking sheets with parchment paper.

4. Spoon the dough (approximately 2 tablespoons of each cookie) on the baking sheets. Bake within 15 minutes, until slightly golden at the borders. Remove from the oven and allow the cookies to remain on the baking sheet for about 20 minutes.

5. For the glaze, combine the powdered sugar, lemon juice, and lemon zest in a small bowl and then stir until smooth.

6. Spoon approximately 1/2-tsp on each cookie and use the back of the spoon to disperse lightly. Allow glaze to harden for about two hours. Pack the biscuits in a decorative jar.

Nutrition:

Calories: 113

Fat: 3.5 g

Carbs: 19 g

Protein: 0 g

18. Peanut Butter Snack Balls

Preparation Time: 10 minutes

Cooking Time: 0 minutes

Servings: 16

Ingredients:

- 1/2 cup chunky peanut butter

- 3 tbsp flax seeds

- 3 tbsp wheat germ

- 1 tbsp honey or agave

- 1/4 cup powdered sugar

Directions:

1. Blend dry ingredients and adding from honey and peanut butter. Mix well and roll into chunks and then conclude by rolling into wheat germ. Serve.

Nutrition:

Calories: 59

Carbs: 8g

Fat: 2g .Protein: 1g

19. Mascarpone Cheesecake with Almond Crust

Preparation Time: 15 minutes

Cooking Time: 1 hour

Servings: 12

Ingredients:

Crust:

- 1/2 cup slivered almonds
- 8 tsp or 2/3 cup graham cracker crumbs
- 2 tbsp sugar
- 1 tbsp salted butter melted

Filling:

- 1 (8-ounce) packages cream cheese, room temperature
- 1 (8-ounce) container mascarpone cheese, room temperature
- 3/4 cup sugar
- 1 tsp fresh lemon juice

- 1 tsp vanilla extract

- 2 large eggs, room temperature

Directions:

1. For the crust, warm the oven to 350 degrees F. You will need a 9-inch pan. Finely grind the almonds, cracker crumbs sugar in a food processor. Put the butter and process until moist crumbs form.

2. Press the almond mixture on the prepared pan's base (maybe not on the edges of the pan). Bake the crust until it's set and start to brown, about 1-2 minutes. Cool. Adjust the temperature to 325 degrees F.

3. For your filling, with an electric mixer, beat the cream cheese, mascarpone cheese, and sugar in a large bowl until smooth, occasionally scraping down the sides of the jar using a rubber spatula.

4. Beat in the lemon juice and vanilla. Put the eggs one at a time, beating until combined after each addition.

5. Pour the cheese mixture on the crust from the pan. Put the pan into a big skillet or Pyrex dish pour enough hot water into the roasting pan to come halfway up the sides of one's skillet.

6. Bake until the middle of the filling moves slightly when the pan is gently shaken, about 1 hour. Transfer the cake to a stand; chill for 1 hour. Refrigerate until the cheesecake is cold, at least eight hours.

7. For the topping, squeeze just a small thick cream in the microwave using a chopped Lindt dark chocolate - afterward, get a Ziplock baggie and cut out a hole at the corner, then pour the melted chocolate into the baggie and used this to decorate the cake!

Nutrition:

Calories: 410

Carbs: 39g

Fat: 26g

Protein: 7g

20. Pizza Kale Chips

Preparation Time: 20 minutes

Cooking Time: 12 hours

Servings: 6

Ingredients:

- 1 tsp dried oregano

- 1 tsp dried marjoram

- 1 tsp garlic powder

- 1 tsp onion powder

- 8 cup kale, leaves from about six stalks, veins removed

- 1 cup raw cashew

- 1/2 cup tomato paste, one small can

- 2 tbsp. nutritional yeast, Lewis labs brewer's yeast buds (from sugar beets)

- 1/2 tsp salt

- 1/4 tsp red pepper flakes

- 1 tsp dried basil

- 1/2 tsp dried rosemary

Directions:

1. Place the cashews in a tub, cover with filtered water and allow the cashews, preferably overnight, to soak refrigerated for at least 2 hours.

2. Drain away the cashew juice. Place the cashews in a meal processor or blender. To only cover the cashews, apply filtered water, and heat until creamy smooth.

3. Stir together the cashew cream in a large mixing bowl with all remaining ingredients except the kale. Stir until the combination is even. Rinse the kale and take the leaves off the fibrous roots. Tear the pieces into "chip" size.

4. Take the kale away with the cashew cream filled with "pizza." You may need to do this a little bit at a time, ensuring that coverage is assured. Dehydrate the kale chips for 12 hours, then cook at 105-115 degrees. Serve.

Nutrition:

Calories: 304

Fat: 17 g

Carbs: 27 g

21. Tuscan Bean Stew

Preparation Time: 10 minutes

Cooking Time: 40 minutes

Servings: 4

Ingredients:

- 1 tbsp. extra virgin olive oil
- 50g red onion, finely chopped
- 30g carrot, peeled and finely chopped
- 30g celery, trimmed and finely chopped
- One garlic clove, finely chopped
- ½ bird's eye chili, finely chopped (optional)
- 1 tsp herbs de Provence
- 200ml vegetable stock
- 1 x 400g tin chopped Italian tomatoes
- 1 tsp tomato purée
- 200g tinned mixed beans
- 50g kale, roughly chopped
- 1 tbsp. roughly chopped parsley

- 40g buckwheat

Directions:

1. Put the oil over low to medium heat in a medium saucepan and fry the onion, carrot, celery, garlic, chili, and herbs gently until the onion is soft but not colored.

2. Stir in stock, tomatoes, and purée tomatoes and carry to boil. Attach the beans and require cooking for 30 minutes. Put the kale and cook for within 5–10 minutes, then add the parsley until tender.

3. In the meantime, cook the buckwheat as instructed by the package, drain, and then serve with stew.

Nutrition:

Calories: 365

Fat: 5 g

Carbs: 67 g

Protein: 16 g

22. Chocolate Nut Truffles

Preparation Time: 10 minutes

Cooking Time: 5 minutes

Servings: 25

Ingredients:

- 1 tbsp. Frangelico or 1 tsp vanilla extract

- 50g hazelnut, roughly chopped

- 175ml double cream

- 200g bar dark chocolate, finely chopped

- Different colored sprinkles and edible glitters

Directions:

1. Put the milk into a tiny saucepan to the boiling level. Take the minced chocolate from the flame and pour it over.

2. Gently whisk the mixture up to clear, then apply the alcohol or coffee extract and the hazelnuts. Cover and put in the fridge for 30 minutes, or until dense but not substantial.

3. Scoop out the mixture's teaspoons and form with your hands into little spheres. Place each of your sprinkles or glitters on different plaques or containers.

4. Roll each truffle to cover in the sprinkles or shimmer, then chill again to firm up. Will keep it refrigerated for one week or freeze without decoration for up to 1 month.

Nutrition:

Calories: 90

Fat: 7 g

Carbs: 5 g

Protein: 1 g

23. Chocolate Balls

Preparation Time: 15 minutes

Cooking Time: 0 minute

Servings: 36

Ingredients:

- 400g can condensed milk

- 1/2 cup desiccated coconut

- 200 grams Arrowroot biscuits crushed

- 3 tablespoons cacao powder

Directions:

1. Mix the broken biscuit, chocolate, and condensed milk to create a sticky consistency. Using a generous mixture tablespoon, shape into balls and wrap in coconut. Chill it before you drink.

Nutrition:

Calories: 121

Fat: 7.8 g

Carbs: 12.9 g .Protein: 2.5 g

24. Vanilla Crème Brule

Preparation Time: 20 minutes

Cooking Time: 30 minutes

Servings: 4

Ingredients:

- 1 cup vanilla sugar, divided
- 6 large egg yolks
- 2 quarts hot water
- 1-quart heavy cream
- 1 vanilla bean split and scraped

Directions:

1. Preheat the oven to 160°C.

2. Place the milk, vanilla bean, and pulp in a medium-high heat saucepan and bring to a boil. Remove from the heat, cover, and allow for 15 minutes of sitting. Remove the vanilla bean and set aside for further use.

3. Whisk 1/2 cup sugar and the egg yolks together in a medium bowl until well mixed until it only begins to lighten in color.

4. Apply the milk, continually mixing, a little at a time. Pour the liquid into six ramekins, then put it in a large cake saucepan or roast pan.

5. Put enough hot water into your saucepan to halfway up the sides of the ramekins. Bake for about 40 to 45 minutes until the crème Brule is set but still trembling in the center.

6. Remove the ramekins from the roasting oven, and cool for at least two hours and up to three days in general.

7. Reserve the Brule cream from the refrigerator for at least 30 minutes before the sugar has browned. Divide the remaining 1/2 cup vanilla sugar equally over the six bowls, then sprinkle uniformly over the bottom.

8. Melt the sugar using a flame, then shape a crispy layer. Enable the crème Brule to sit for 5 minutes or more before serving.

Nutrition:

Calories: 400

Carbs: 26 g

Fat: 32 g

Protein: 3 g

25. Healthy Coffee Cookies

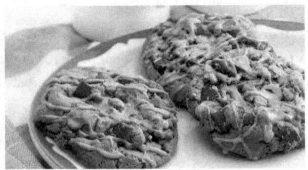

Preparation time: 15 – 20 minutes

Cooking time: 12 - 15 minutes

Servings: 20

Ingredients:

For dry ingredients:

- ½ cup cocoa, unsweetened
- 6 tablespoons all-purpose flour
- ½ cup whole-wheat flour
- ¾ tablespoon finely ground coffee beans or instant coffee
- ½ teaspoon baking soda
- ¾ teaspoon ground cinnamon
- ¼ teaspoon kosher salt

For wet ingredients:

- 3 small eggs, lightly beaten

- ¼ cup nonfat or low-fat plain Greek yogurt

- ½ tablespoon olive oil

- ½ + 1/8 cup blueberries

- ½ ripe banana

- ¼ cup honey

- 1 teaspoon pure vanilla extract

- ¼ cup dark or semi-sweet chocolate chips

Directions:

1. Preheat the oven to 350°F. Prepare a baking sheet by oiling with nonstick cooking spray. Set it aside.

2. Combine all the dry ingredients, i.e., whole-wheat flour, all-purpose flour, cocoa, cinnamon, salt, baking soda, and coffee in a mixing bowl.

3. Place banana in a microwave-safe bowl and cook on high for about 50 seconds. Mash the banana and add into a bowl. Also, add eggs, yogurt, oil, honey, and vanilla. Mix until well incorporated.

4. Pour the wet ingredients into the dry ingredients and mix until just combined, making sure not to over-mix. Add chocolate chips and blueberries and fold gently.

5. Make 20 equal portions of the mixture and place it on the baking sheet. It should be approximately 1-½

tablespoons per portion. Press the cookies lightly. You can use a fork to do so.

6. Put the baking sheet in your oven and bake within about 12 – 14 minutes. When the cookies are ready, they will be visibly hard around the edges.

7. Cool on the baking sheet for 10 minutes. Loosen the cookies by pushing a metal spatula underneath the cookies. Transfer onto a wire rack. Serve.

Nutrition:

Calories 60

Fat 1.5 g

Carbohydrate 11 g

Protein 2 g

26. Strawberry Oatmeal Bars

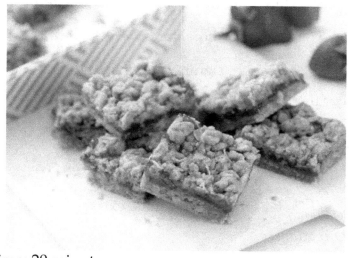

Preparation time: 20 minutes

Cooking time: 35 – 40 minutes

Servings: 8

Ingredients:

For strawberry bars:

- ½ cup old-fashioned rolled oats
- 3 tablespoons light brown sugar
- 1/8 teaspoon kosher salt
- 1 cup small-diced strawberries, divided

- ½ tablespoon fresh lemon juice

- 6 tablespoons white whole wheat flour

- 1/8 teaspoon ground ginger

- 3 tablespoons unsalted butter, melted

- ½ teaspoon cornstarch

- 3 teaspoons granulated sugar, divided

For the vanilla glaze: Optional

- ¼ cup powdered sugar sifted

- ½ tablespoon milk

- ¼ teaspoon pure vanilla extract

Directions:

1. Preheat the oven to 350°F. Prepare a small square or rectangular baking pan by lining it with a large parchment paper sheet such that the extra sheet is hanging from 2 opposite sides.

2. Add oats, brown sugar, flour, salt, and ginger into a bowl and stir well. Put butter and mix.

3. Take out about 4 tablespoons of the mixture into a bowl and set it aside. Transfer the rest of the mixture into the baking pan. Press it well onto the bottom of the baking pan.

4. Spread ½ cup chopped strawberries over the crust — dust cornstarch over it. Drizzle the lemon juice over the strawberries. Sprinkle 1 ½ teaspoons sugar.

5. Spread remaining strawberries and 1 ½ teaspoons sugar over it. Scatter the retained crumb mixture on top. Put the baking dish in your oven and bake for about 30 – 35 minutes or until golden brown on top. Take out the baking dish and place it on the wire rack to cool.

6. Meanwhile, make the glaze. For this, add powdered sugar, milk, and vanilla into a bowl and whisk well. Lift the bars along with the parchment paper and place it on your cutting board. Pour glaze on top. Cut into 8 equal bars and serve.

Nutrition:

Calories 100

Fat 5 g

Carbohydrate 14 g

Protein 2 g

27. Parsley Cheese Balls

Preparation time: 15 minutes

Cooking time: 0 minutes

Servings: 12

Ingredients:

- ¼ cup shredded, Kraft 2% milk sharp cheddar cheese
- 1 package (8 ounces) Philadelphia Neufchatel cheese, softened
- ½ tablespoon finely chopped green onion
- ½ tablespoon finely chopped red pepper
- ¼ cup finely chopped parsley
- 1 teaspoon Dijon mustard
- 6 stalks celery, cut each into 4 equal pieces crosswise
- 60 whole-wheat Ritz crackers

Directions:

1. Add Neufchatel and cheddar cheeses into a bowl. Beat with an electric hand mixer until well combined. Stir in green onion, red pepper, and Dijon mustard.

2. Place the bowl in the refrigerator for an hour. Split the batter into 12 equal portions and shape into balls.

3. Place parsley on a plate. Dredge the balls in parsley. Place on a plate. Chill until use. Each serving should consist of a cheese ball with 2 pieces parsley and 5 Ritz crackers.

Nutrition:

Calories 130

Fat 7 g

Carbohydrate 12 g

Protein 3 g

28. Baked Kale Chips

Preparation time: 10 minutes

Cooking time: 10 minutes

Servings: 3

Ingredients:

- ½ bunch kale (stiff stems and ribs discarded), torn into bite-size pieces
- Salt to taste
- ½ tablespoon olive oil
- Spices of your choice to flavor (optional)

Directions:

1. Preheat the oven to 350°F. Dry the kale using a salad spinner. Place kale on the baking sheet. Trickle oil over it. Sprinkle salt over the kale and spread it evenly.

2. Put the baking sheet in your oven and bake within about 12 – 14 minutes or until crisp. Cool completely and serve. Store the leftovers in an airtight container.

Nutrition:

Calories 58

Fat 2.8 g

Carbohydrate 7.6 g

Protein 2.5 g

Chapter 2. Sauces & Dips

29. Sweet and Savory Cherry Compote

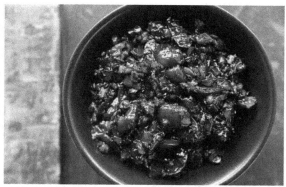

Preparation time: 15 minutes

Cooking time: 10 minutes

Servings: 6

Ingredients:

- 2 1/2 cups pitted sweet cherries, slice into quarter

- 1 cup walnuts, thinly chopped

- 2 tablespoons red onion, diced

- 3 tablespoons extra virgin olive oil

- ¼ cup port red wine or cherry juice

- ¼ tsp sea salt

- 1 tablespoon honey

- 1 teaspoon rosemary, fresh

- ¼ tsp black pepper, ground

Directions:

1. Add the extra virgin olive oil into a large skillet and sauté the red onion over medium heat until the red onion is soft and tender and beginning to turn golden around the edges, about 3 minutes. Be sure to stir the onions occasionally, so the onion cooks evenly.

2. Add the cherries, walnuts, and rosemary to the skillet and continue to stir until the cherries become tender about 5 minutes. Add in the seasonings and adjust the amount to fit your taste.

3. Pour in the red wine or cherry juice along with the honey. Allow the cherries to cook in the wine simmering until the cherries are soft and the liquid has become thick with a syrup-like texture.

Nutrition:

Calories: 120

Carbs: 21g

Fat: 3g

Protein: 3g

30. Cilantro Lime Sauce

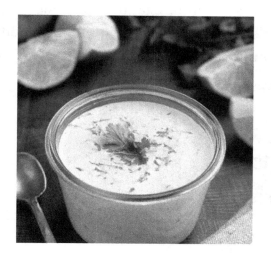

Preparation time: 15 minutes

Cooking time: 0 minutes

Servings: 2

Ingredients:

- ½ cup Soy yogurt, plain
- ½ tsp Black pepper, ground
- 1 tablespoon Lime juice
- 1 teaspoon Lime Zest
- 6 tablespoons cilantro, chopped
- ½ tbsp Extra virgin olive oil
- ½ tsp Sea salt

Directions:

1. Puree all of the cilantro-lime sauce ingredients in a blender or food processor until smooth. Serve the sauce immediately, or store in the fridge for up to a week.

Nutrition:

Calories: 95

Carbs: 1g

Fat: 10g

Protein: 0g

31. Greek Tzatziki Sauce

Preparation time: 15 minutes

Cooking time: 0 minutes

Servings: 12

Ingredients:

- 1 cup Soy yogurt, plain
- 1 & ½ cup English cucumber, grated
- 1 tablespoon Extra virgin olive oil
- 2 cloves garlic, minced
- 2 teaspoons Lemon juice
- ½ tsp Sea salt
- 2 teaspoons parsley, chopped
- 2 teaspoons Dill, chopped

Directions:

1. In a kitchen, a bowl whisks together all of the ingredients, excluding the cucumber. Put the grated cucumber in a clean towel, and squeeze it over the sink to remove as much liquid as possible.

2. Add the cucumber to the bowl, stirring it together to combine. Serve immediately, or store in the fridge for up to four to five days.

Nutrition:

Calories: 25

Carbs: 3g

Fat: 0g

32. Green Enchilada Sauce

Preparation time: 15 minutes

Cooking time: 12 minutes

Servings: 6

Ingredients:

- ½ cup of water
- ½ cup cashews, raw
- 2 cups cilantro, chopped
- 1 jalapeno, chopped
- 7 oz green chilies, canned
- 1 & ½ tsp apple cider vinegar
- 1 teaspoon of sea salt

Directions:

1. Soak or dip the cashews, cover them with water and allow them to sit covered for 6 to 12 hours, or simmer them on the stove in water for 15 minutes. Drain off the water and add the cashews to a blender.

2. Into the blender, add the remaining ingredients, and blend the enchilada sauce until it is completely smooth.

Use the green enchilada sauce immediately or store it in the refrigerator for up to a week.

Nutrition:

Calories: 25

Carbs: 3g

Fat: 2g

33. Jalapeno Pineapple Aioli

Preparation time: 15 minutes

Cooking time: 0 minutes

Servings: 12

Ingredients:

- 1 1/2 cups mayonnaise made with olive oil
- 3 tablespoons onion, minced
- ¼ cup cilantro, chopped
- 1 jalapeno, minced
- ½ cup canned pineapple, minced
- 1 clove garlic, minced
- 2 tablespoons pineapple juice from the can
- 1 tablespoon lime juice
- ½ tsp sea salt
- ½ tsp red pepper flakes
- 1 teaspoon lime zest

Directions:

1. If you want a chunky sauce, add everything to a bowl and stir it. For a smooth, creamy sauce, pulse everything together in a blender until creamy. Serve the jalapeno pineapple aioli immediately or store in the fridge for up to a week.

Nutrition:

Calories: 172

Carbs: 6g

Fat: 16g

Protein: 1g

34. Awesome Sauce

Preparation time: 15 minutes

Cooking time: 3 minutes

Servings: 8

Ingredients:

- ½ cup Mayonnaise made with olive oil
- 1 teaspoon Sea salt
- 2 teaspoons Mustard
- 1 cup Onion, diced
- 1 tablespoon Extra virgin olive oil
- 2 tablespoons parsley, chopped
- 1 tablespoon Chives, chopped
- 1 tablespoon Dill, chopped
- ¼ tsp Black pepper, ground

Directions:

1. Add the onions and olive oil to a skillet, allowing them to sauté until slightly translucent, about three minutes over medium-high heat.

2. In a blender, combine all of the awesome sauce ingredients, except for the chopped herbs. Continue to pulse until creamy, and then gently stir in the chopped herbs. Serve the sauce immediately, or store in the fridge for up to a week.

Nutrition:

Calories: 80

Carbs: 1g

Fat: 7g

Protein: 0g

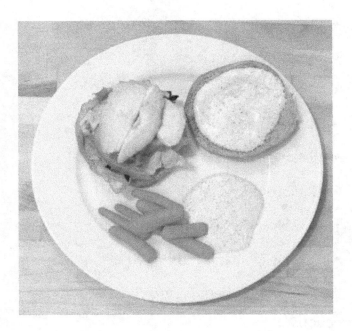

35. Vegan Hollandaise Sauce

Preparation time: 15 minutes

Cooking time: 0 minutes

Servings: 8

Ingredients:

- 1 cup Mayonnaise made with olive oil (vegan)
- 1 teaspoon Lemon juice
- 3 tablespoons vegan butter, melted
- ½ tsp Turmeric, ground
- ¼ tsp Cayenne pepper
- ¼ tsp Black pepper, ground

Directions:

1. Add all of the vegan Hollandaise sauce ingredients to a small saucepan and cook it over medium heat until heated through. Be careful not to allow the Hollandaise sauce to boil. Remove from heat and use hot. Enjoy the sauce immediately, or store it for up to a week.

Nutrition:

Calories: 67

Carbs: 0g Fat: 7g Protein: 1g

36. Vegan Cheese Sauce

Preparation time: 15 minutes

Cooking time: 10 minutes

Servings: 6

Ingredients:

- 1 yellow summer squash, sliced
- 1 sweet potato, medium, peeled and diced
- 4 cloves garlic, minced
- 1 onion, diced
- 2 cups vegetable broth
- ¼ cup nutritional yeast
- 1 & ½ tsp sea salt
- ¼ tsp mustard powder
- ¼ tsp paprika
- ¼ tsp black pepper, ground

Directions:

1. Add the diced potato to a pot of boiling water, and allow it to cook until tender, about seven to ten minutes.

2. Meanwhile, sauté the onion and yellow squash in the vegetable broth. Slowly add the vegetable broth as needed, using about one-quarter of a cup at a time and adding more as needed.

3. Add in the minced garlic, and sauté until it becomes aromatic about 3 minutes. Add the cooked onion, squash, and potato into a blender with the remaining vegetable broth and all of the seasonings.

4. Combine at high speed until the sauce is incredibly smooth. Feel free to add more broth to adjust the thickness to your preference.

Nutrition:

Calories: 37

Carbs: 6g

Fat: 1g

Protein: 3g

37. Teriyaki Sauce

Preparation time: 15 minutes

Cooking time: 5 minutes

Servings: 6

Ingredients:

- ¼ cup tamari sauce
- 1 & ¼ cup water, divided
- 2 tablespoons cornstarch
- ¼ cup honey
- ½ tsp ginger, grated
- 1 clove garlic, minced

Directions:

1. Mix the one-quarter cup of water and cornstarch in a small bowl. Set the slurry aside.

2. In a saucepan, add the remaining water and the tamari sauce, honey, garlic, and ginger. While stirring, cook over medium heat until it reaches a simmer.

3. Add the cornstarch slurry into the saucepan while whisking, and continue to cook the sauce until thickened, about seven minutes.

4. Remove the easy teriyaki sauce from the stove and allow it to sit for five to ten minutes before using, to let it to finish thickening.

Nutrition:

Calories: 15

Carbs: 2g

Fat: 0g

Protein: 1g

38. Thai Peanut Sauce

Preparation time: 15 minutes

Cooking time: 0 minutes

Servings: 6

Ingredients:

- ½ cup peanut butter, natural
- 1 teaspoon honey
- ½ cup of soy milk
- 2 tablespoons tamari sauce
- ½ tsp ginger, grated
- 1 tablespoon lime juice
- 1 teaspoon sriracha sauce
- 1 clove garlic, minced

Directions:

1. Add all of the Thai peanut sauce ingredients into a blender and combine until smooth, and the garlic is well combined. Use the peanut sauce immediately or store it in the fridge for up to a week.

Nutrition:

Calories: 40

Carbs: 3g

Fat: 2g

Protein: 1g

39. Tasty Vegan Gravy

Preparation time: 15 minutes

Cooking time: 17 minutes

Servings: 6

Ingredients:

- 2 cloves garlic, minced

- ½ tsp sea salt

- 4 ounces mushrooms, sliced

- 1 onion, diced

- 1 tablespoon extra-virgin olive oil

- 1 Yukon gold potato, peeled and diced

- 1 cup of water

- 2 tablespoons tamari sauce

- ¼ tsp black pepper, ground

Directions:

1. Sauté your onion in the extra virgin olive oil until tender and translucent, about 5 minutes, and then add in the mushrooms and garlic. Continue stirring until the garlic is fragrant and golden, about 1 to 2 minutes.

2. Into the skillet, add the Yukon Gold potato, water, and tamari sauce, allowing it to reach a boil over medium-high heat.

3. Reduce the stove to medium and cover the steel skillet with a lid. Allow the potatoes to cook until they are tender, about 10 minutes.

4. Carefully pour the potatoes, mushrooms, and other skillet contents into a blender along with the seasonings.

5. Instead of the plastic cap, use a towel to cover the opening, which will allow steam to escape while also keeping the contents in the blender.

6. Blend the contents at high speed until completely smooth and creamy. Adjust the seasoning to your taste and enjoy.

Nutrition:

Calories: 31

Carbs: 6g

Fat: 0g

Protein: 2g

Chapter 3. Juices & Smoothies

40. Kale Kiwi Smoothie

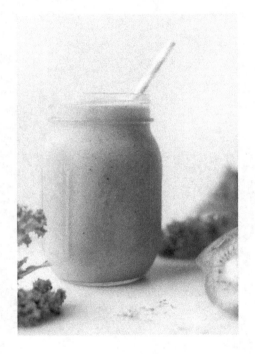

Preparation Time: 10 minutes

Cooking Time: 0 minutes

Servings: 1

Ingredients:

- 1 cup kale, chopped

- 2 Apples

- 3 Kiwis

- 1 tablespoon flax seeds

- 1 tablespoon royal jelly

- 1 cup crushed ice

Directions:

1. Put all of the fixings into a blender and cover them with water. Blitz until smooth. Serve.

Nutrition:

Calories: 250

Carbs: 35g

Fat: 1g

Protein: 15g

41. Salad Smoothie

Preparation Time: 10 minutes

Cooking Time: 0 minutes

Servings: 1

Ingredients:

- 1 cup arugula
- ½ cucumber
- 1/2 small red onion
- 2 tablespoons Parsley
- 2 tablespoons lemon juice
- 1 cup crushed ice
- 1 tbsp. olive oil or cumin oil

Directions:

1. Put all the fixing into a blender with some water and blitz until smooth. Add ice to make your smoothie refreshing.

Nutrition:

Calories: 80

Carbs: 20g

Fat: 0g

Protein: 1g

42. Avocado Kale Smoothie

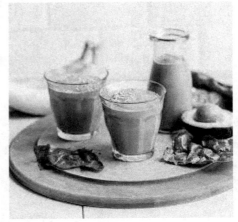

Preparation Time: 10 minutes

Cooking Time: 0 minutes

Servings: 1

Ingredients:

- 1 cup kale
- ½ avocado
- 1 cup cucumber
- 1 celery stalk
- 1 tbsp. chia seeds
- 1 cup crushed ice
- 1 tbsp. spirulina

Directions:

1. Put all of the fixings into a blender and add in enough water to cover them. Process until smooth, serve, and enjoy.

Nutrition:

Calories: 377

Carbs: 0g

Fat: 0g

Protein: 0g

43. Kale Banana Apple Smoothie

Preparation Time: 10 minutes

Cooking Time: 0 minutes

Servings: 1

Ingredients:

- 1 cup kale
- 2 apples
- 3/4 avocado
- 1 banana
- 1 cup crushed ice

Directions:

1. Put all of the fixings into a blender and process until smooth. Serve and enjoy.

Nutrition:

Calories: 150

Carbs: 29g

Fat: 0g

Protein: 2g

44. Kale Cucumber Apple Smoothie

Preparation Time: 10 minutes

Cooking Time: 0 minutes

Servings: 1

Ingredients:

- 1 cup kale
- 2 apples
- 1 avocado
- 1 lime
- 1/4 cup raspberries
- 1 cucumber
- 1 cup crushed ice

Directions:

1. Put all of the fixings into the blender with enough water to cover them and blitz until smooth.

Nutrition:

Calories: 120

Carbs: 0g

Fat: 0g

Protein: 5g

45. Grapefruit Kale Smoothie

Preparation Time: 10 minutes

Cooking Time: 0 minutes

Servings: 1

Ingredients:

- 1 large grapefruit
- 1 apple
- 1 cup watercress
- 2 kale leaves
- 1 tbsp. dill (optional)
- 1 cup crushed ice

Directions:

1. Put all of the fixings into a blender and add enough water to cover them. Process until creamy and smooth.

Nutrition:

Calories: 233

Carbs: 37g

Fat: 4g .Protein: 16g

46. Pear Cilantro Smoothie

Preparation Time: 10 minutes

Cooking Time: 0 minutes

Servings: 1

Ingredients:

- 1 cup parsley leaves

- 1 pear

- 3/4 avocado

- ½ lemon - juice

- 1 tbsp. chopped cilantro

- 1 cup crushed ice

Directions:

1. Process all of the fixings into a blender with water to cover them. Add a few ice cubes and enjoy.

Nutrition:

Calories: 413

Carbs: 97g .Fat: 3g .Protein: 3g

Conclusion

Congratulations! You now know how to follow the Sirtfood diet diligently and lose weight healthily and consistently.

There are several diets out there. Dieting has become an industry of its own, with videos, books, blogs, and all sorts of diet pills, supplements, and other items accessible to customers. At the same time, Western nations are becoming more health-conscious and overweight, and, as a result, there is a rising demand for information on diets and items related to weight loss. However, what's not much of it is solid, useful information about how to successfully diet-that is, how to effectively lose weight and keep it off.

Anyone can lose weight by following one of the many fad diets available. Still, these diets have a few fatal flaws. They generally do not provide you with a nutritionally healthy diet; they're not intended for anything other than short-term weight loss and, perhaps worst of all, they generally do not provide you with any sleep.

However, you don't need fad diet plans or diet pills to eat effectively; you need the right details on what to do and what to avoid when you're trying to lose weight. The SirtFood diet is 70-80 percent raw and also contains the following:

Motivation: If you are not motivated to lose weight and improve your health, you probably won't be successful regardless of what kind of diet you follow. It needs the self-discipline to avoid food mistakes, and to get enough exercise, you need to lose weight and keep it off. Without that, nothing is going to work for you in the long run.

Water: Drinking plenty of water is something you can do in the first place because it is so crucial to good health. Drinking eight or more cups of water a day helps your digestive system work more efficiently, helping you lose weight, and drinking water also helps you feel full; in many cases, you may be thirsty when you feel hungry. Drink a glass of water when you're feeling hungry and make a point of getting a glass before meals; you might be shocked by how much less you consume by mealtimes.

Daily Drill: We all know that we need regular exercise, especially if we're trying to lose weight. If you're not getting some form of exercise regularly, try starting small with a half-hour walk every day and work your way up to more intensive exercise and longer workouts. Usually, you'll get the best results with half an hour to 45 minutes of exercise at least three or four days a week. Even if you don't have a lot of spare time on your day, try to put in a little physical exercise whenever you can, take the stairs instead of the elevator, walk to the store instead of driving, or to take a cab, and so on – every little bit helps you lose excess weight and keep it off.

Good, Nutritionally Balanced Diets: We all have an excellent idea of what we should eat; fresh vegetables and fruit, whole grains, small amounts of healthy fats like olive oil, fish, and other lean meats. It is more important to keep your mind clear: refined flours, sugar, processed foods, and any food or beverage filled with preservatives and other artificial ingredients. Get into the habit of carefully reading food labels and, if possible, cook your food with fresh ingredients instead of purchasing pre-made packaged food. It's OK to get a little out of your diet once in a while. But most of the time, you need to stick to the plan.

When you get used to eating healthy, you will find that you quickly lose your appetite for less nutritious choices, and, combined with daily exercise, it will make it easier to stay away from the weight you've gained.

CPSIA information can be obtained
at www.ICGtesting.com
Printed in the USA
LVHW081124080421
683843LV00011B/772